I0705503

Having Your Own Back

Finding Motivation and Creating Healthy Mindsets

A.R.

© **Copyright 2021 - All rights reserved.**

The content contained within this book may not be reproduced, duplicated or transmitted without direct written permission from the author or the publisher.

Under no circumstances will any blame or legal responsibility be held against the publisher, or author, for any damages, reparation, or monetary loss due to the information contained within this book, either directly or indirectly.

Legal Notice:

This book is copyright protected. It is only for personal use. You cannot amend, distribute, sell, use, quote or paraphrase any part, or the content within this book, without the consent of the author or publisher.

<u>Disclaimer Notice:</u>

Please note the information contained within this document is for educational and entertainment purposes only. All effort has been executed to present accurate, up to date, reliable, complete information. No warranties of any kind are declared or implied. Readers acknowledge that the author is not engaged in the rendering of legal, financial, medical or professional advice. The content within this book has been derived from various sources. Please consult a licensed professional before attempting any techniques outlined in this book.

By reading this document, the reader agrees that under no circumstances is the author responsible for any losses, direct or indirect, that are incurred as a result of the use of the information contained within this document, including, but not limited to, errors, omissions, or inaccuracies.

Table of Contents

Table of Contents 4

Introduction 5

Chapter 1: Have Your Own Back 12

Chapter 2: Pointless Comparisons 23

Chapter 3: Abundance vs Scarcity 33

Chapter 4: Appreciate Reality 45

Chapter 5: Self-Motivation and Your Goals 55

Chapter 6: Failure 67

Conclusion 77

References 83

Introduction

"If you believe it will work out, you will see opportunities. If you do not believe it will work out, you will see obstacles." - Wayne Dyer

Have you heard the story of a wise old man who lived on the outskirts of a village and served as a counselor to the villagers. People would often walk up to his house, asking for advice on important matters and sharing their problems with him at length. The wise man was never bothered by this, as he loved helping anyone he met, regardless of their reputation.

After a year of listening to their problems, the man had noticed a pattern in his fellow villagers. He noticed that every week, they would complain about the same thing. So one day, he invited everyone to his house to share a meal. Towards the end of the night, the wise man decided to tell a joke.

Everyone roared with laughter at this display. A few minutes later, the wise man repeated the joke to everyone, but this time, only a few people even smiled. Five minutes later, he repeated the same joke. This time, no one smiled or made a sound. He went quiet for a moment, as if he was thinking of what to say next. He then smiled his same warm smile and addressed the stoic crowd gathered in his home. "You can not laugh at the same joke over and over. So why do you choose to cry about the same problem?"

Without realizing it, this is how many of us spend our lives. We try to deal with our problems the same way every time, and then complain when things do not go our way. We give up because we start to tell ourselves that we are failures. We convince ourselves that we are unworthy because we could not overcome an obstacle. How often do we deprive ourselves of success due to the fear of failure?

When we have goals we want to reach, it is sometimes easy to get lost along the way. It can be easy to be overburdened by obstacles that blind us from reaching our destination. For example, visualize yourself walking down a narrow path. Suddenly, you come across a huge boulder blocking your way. There is no way to get over it, nor can you see what is behind it. You try to push the large rock out of the way, but it will not budge. You realize that there is no way to get past, so you give up and head home. On your way back, you are lost in your thoughts and begin to wallow in self-pity. This causes your vision to narrow and become skewed, and you miss the alternate route that has now appeared on the side of the road.

In life, if we do not have the motivation, it is easy to give up midway. We promise ourselves we will try again, but when we do, we repeat the same process over. We have goals and dreams, but we have no plan of action to achieve them. We never leave our comfort zones and stay stuck in the same loop for years to come.

Our mind plays a major role in whether or not we achieve these goals. When we encounter problems, we allow ourselves to dwell on them for far too long. The longer we linger, the more we convince ourselves to give up. We allow our intrusive thoughts to control us and our actions. We also let them fog our minds, making it hard to focus on what we want out of life.

This book aims to break those cycles by teaching you important lessons that you can use for the rest of your life. I will aim to push you to your limits but not break them. In the first chapter, I will highlight what it means to be a leader for yourself and others. I will also show you simple techniques you can use to boost self-esteem, something crucial to staying motivated.

Before we continue, I would like to highlight how important it is for you not to try and complete too many things at once. I would suggest rereading and applying each chapter before attempting the next. Do not overburden yourself, as this is a common way to fail. Failing before you fully grasp these concepts can have the opposite of the intended results. If you fail before you have learned to deal with failure, you are more likely to give up prematurely. So I urge you to take it easy and allow yourself to move at a pace that is comfortable.

The second chapter teaches you about comparisons and why they are dangerous. We will also touch on emotions and how to control them. This chapter is crucial in improving the way you see yourself.

In chapter three, we talk about mindsets. Having the right type of mindset will determine how far you go and what you can achieve in life.

Next, in chapter four we attempt to define reality. As Alan Watts once said, "What is reality? Obviously, no one can say because it isn't words. It isn't material, that's just an idea. Reality *is*." What he is trying to say here is: reality is here, and it's now. We will learn how to appreciate everything around us and everything we have accomplished so far. Read further to find out why this is so important in our journey of self-discovery.

Once you are able to apply these ideas, move on to chapter five, where we learn how to find out where our happiness lies, and what we truly crave in life. We learn how to self-motivate, and finally, how to set appropriate goals for ourselves.

Last, but definitely not the least, we talk about failure. In this chapter, we uncover the secret to dealing with failure and how to recover from it. We will also explore problem solving skills and how they can help us in everyday life.

By the end of this book, you should be motivated enough to create and achieve your goals. You will also have increased knowledge of self and a newfound admiration. There is no doubt that you will soon feel more energized and generally happier.

When you desire something from the depths of your heart, there is little that can stop you from achieving it. It is for that reason that we all have to dig deep within ourselves to find where our happiness lies. We will not spend any more time following dreams that are tailored for another person.

To get the most out of this book, I suggest reading it with an open mind. You must have the willingness to learn, but above all, you must be willing to change. Just seeing information written on a page will make no difference to you and your life, it is what you do with the knowledge that really matters.

Self-motivation is what helps us to keep moving forward. Motivation can come from many different sources. It can be internal or external; it can arise from love or the desire to seek wealth. To discover what spurs your motivation, you must first discover yourself.

Later in the book, we will take a trip to find out what motivates you, and how to activate it when necessary. Your self-motivation is what will help keep moving you forward, even in the face of adversity. When you are ready to quit, your self-motivation is what will stop you. So, by learning the trigger of what motivates us, we can get through many hardships, and reach even the hardest goals.

Becoming self-motivated is not something that happens overnight. After reading this book, you will not suddenly wake up the next morning with a need to take over the world. Remember to take it one step at a time. Your self-motivation skills should build over time so they can become a way of life.

It is crucial to the process that you follow the techniques and suggestions within this book every day. When you practice something every day, you are essentially training yourself to adopt that practice as a habit. Once it becomes a habit, it will be natural for you to do without extra thought. There will come a time when you won't even have to remind yourself to do these things.

If you find *Looking Out for Number One* helpful, feel free to share your knowledge with your friends and colleagues. Remember, you should always surround yourself with like-minded and positive people, as they can influence your life in many ways.

So, without wasting any more time, let's get started. I hope the information I have provided will help you as much as it has helped me.

Chapter 1

Have Your Own Back

"You have power over your mind - not outside events. Realize this, and you will find strength." - Marcus Aurelius

Having a support system in place is extremely important. However, your number one fan should always be yourself. Would you like to be held up, or would you like to hold yourself up? In this chapter, we cover the importance of showing up for you, and how it can improve life.

Whenever we have a problem, we tend to turn to our support systems for help. Family, friends, and colleagues all make up our support systems. They are great to have, but we sometimes forget that they are human and will not be available at all times. So, what happens when they are unavailable to assist us? Without an inner support system, it's easy to become annoyed and even resentful if they are not there during a time of need.

By building yourself up to be self-reliant, you are ensuring that you will be able to get through anything, even when you have no one but yourself.

You also teach yourself that no one owes you the courtesy of being there for you. You can not blame other people if something happens because they were not available to assist you. Most importantly, you are teaching yourself that you should not make yourself readily available to anyone who needs you at any time, and that is self-care.

If you find it hard to support yourself, simply think about the person you love most in this world. Picture them in your situation and think about how you would assist them. If you would offer them advice, then gently offer the same advice to yourself. Be your own best friend.

Remember, being there for yourself is more than just practicing self-care rituals. You need enough self-knowledge to know when you start to struggle, stress out, or when motivation starts to decline. You also have to know yourself well enough to understand what you need and when you need it.

- Embrace your flaws. They make you who you are. They are the reason for your uniqueness. Be willing to accept yourself for the way you are.

- Learn to say no. Say no to people and things who no longer contribute positively to your life. Learn to stay away from those who drain your mental energy. By saying no to them, you are saying yes to yourself. That's a great way to have your own back.

- Set healthy boundaries. Never allow another person to disrespect you or your space. Take the time to get to know yourself so you can understand the type of boundaries you need to set. Never feel guilty for believing in your values, and defend them unapologetically.

- Have some alone time. It is necessary to give yourself some space whenever you can. Use this time to get to know yourself and listen to your inner voice. It will help to uncover what it is you truly crave from life. Your needs might change over time, so it is important to check in regularly.

- Have fun! Doing things you enjoy will ensure that you are giving yourself the chance to be happy. Do at least one fun task every day.

If one of your life goals is to become a leader or hold a position of power, you need to learn how to manage yourself before anything else. Leaders can be the determining factor in whether a company will experience success or failure. This concept applies to our daily lives, as well. If you have no sense of leadership, it's easy to find yourself living on auto-pilot. It means losing out on opportunities and success. Your list of goals remains incomplete because you lack the skill to strive for them. Lack of self-discipline leads to procrastination and low-quality results.

Leadership is applied in all aspects of life, not just in business. Some of the most important places we should be practicing our leadership skills can include:

- At home, where your heart is your domain. You need to have control over your home at all times or be able to share that responsibility with someone who has similar values. Get on top of things before they become an issue. Your home is your safe space, so always keep it in order. Do your chores without having to be reminded, and fix things before they get worse.

- Work, where the secret to becoming a great leader is to lead by example, even if you are not in a leadership position. Prove to yourself and your colleagues that you are worthy of being a leader. You can do this by helping a colleague with a project, be friendly to everyone, especially those in lower positions, and doing slightly more than what is required of you each day.

- Platonic and romantic relationships, as they both require the same amount of effort. Always hold yourself accountable and stay away from the blame game. Understand that investing in your friends and loved ones at all times, not just the beginning, is the secret to successful relationships. The concept of the honeymoon phase is just a myth. That initial attraction only disappears when we get lazy and stop investing. Relationships are like plants that need a lot of resources to survive. Once you stop nurturing them, they die.

- Your physical and mental health, because without a healthy body and mind, all the money in the world will be of no use to you. Make sure you are taking care of your body by exercising regularly and eating healthy food. Take care of your mind by meditating and relaxing. It is the ultimate test of leadership skills, as the self is the hardest person to lead.

- Once you have taken care of the other aspects, it becomes easier to manage your finances with purpose. Whether you realize it or not, you probably know of at least one wealthier person who has filed for bankruptcy, or a less well-off person who enjoys life vigorously. It all boils down to how well you can manage with what you have. Ask yourself if you are saving enough for the future and those unexpected emergencies? Are you spending what you can afford without relying on borrowed money? Have you drafted a living will? If not, today is always a great time to start putting together budgets that better suit your finance

Qualities of a Leader

A true leader can control the way they think. Most leaders have an overall positive mindset. They think with clear minds and can make the best decisions. Leaders know that negative thoughts can poison the mind and spread like wildfire. One negative idea can lead to a flurry of intrusive thinking. Controlling your mind and the way you think can be the deciding factor between success and failure. Leaders never wait to be told what to do, they stay active and take the initiative. Leaders have trained themselves to spot opportunities and grab them. If there are no opportunities, they create them! It is important to work smart, not hard. Those in charge always have their minds set on the bigger picture, thereby making it easier for them to prioritize their days and lives. If you can organize your daily activities with a healthy mix of work, rest, and fun, then you are well on your way to becoming a good leader.

A leader who is only in it for what they get out of it usually lacks the confidence and trust of those they lead. A true leader is not self-serving and lacks the need to be glorified by their peers. Leaders ooze so much confidence that gaining it from external sources holds little to no weight. When you lead without focusing on what you could earn, you gain so much more. You gain the trust and support of those around you, and you also produce better results because of your mindset.

A true leader understands that they do not know everything there is to know. Leaders never stop learning. The best leader is one who can learn from a variety of sources. Leaders are also capable of handling failure with ease. When a leader fails, they see it as nothing more than a learning curve. They use the experience to improve themselves and come back with a better performance. Never allow yourself to get to a point where you stop learning, for that is when you truly fail. You should be able to set your ego aside and allow others to teach you things you might not know. Learn how to listen when others are speaking, and don't interrupt them in the middle of a conversation. Wait until it's your turn, and then raise your concerns. Never allow yourself to be rude to other people under any circumstances. If debates get heated, simply reschedule and give everybody a chance to cool off.

The Importance of Self-Esteem

Self-esteem is an important aspect of being a leader. Without belief in yourself, it is almost impossible to get others to believe in you. You need people to believe in you and trust you before they would be willing to follow you. The idea is to create a healthy sense of self-esteem. If your self-esteem is too low, you will have a negative mindset and be incapable of successfully leading yourself and other people. If you have developed high self-esteem, you might become too self-absorbed, and eventually unteachable.

A healthy level of self-esteem allows you the opportunity to lead with confidence while simultaneously not being afraid of acknowledging your flaws and improving them. Self-esteem helps you believe in yourself, giving you the boost you need to make risky decisions and set high goals. It also means that you are less likely to feel threatened by other people, and instead, you will lead them and encourage them to grow.

Low levels of self-esteem can hold you back in life. If you don't believe in your abilities and feel like you are not enough, you are more likely to quit before you even try. Having a healthy self-image will give you the confidence you need to strive forward. Believe in yourself, your willingness to make things happen, and tackle each challenge with positivity. These are traits a leader should possess.

If you find yourself suffering from negative thinking and fear, you might have a low sense of self-worth. Below, we look at ways to build healthy self-esteem and reap the benefits of feeling more healthy and positive.

Our minds are powerful tools. Our negative mindsets can have a profound impact on our daily lives. The amount of damage it does depends on how much of it we have already begun to believe. A simple way to deal with this is to take a journal and write down all of your negative thoughts. Next to each negative statement, write down a positive one. Whenever you find yourself thinking negatively again, remind yourself that it is not true and repeat the positive affirmations. A lifetime of negative thinking may take a while to remedy, but always keep trying. If you slip up, all you have to do is restart the process. You might even find methods that work better for you, so keep searching. Surround yourself with people who have empathy, supportive people, and are fearless. Avoid relationships that make you feel bad about yourself or other people and stick with those who are kind. Reaching for your goals and working hard every day is necessary, but rest is too. Give yourself a break and remember to decompress. Take a warm bath, have some unadulterated fun, or simply do nothing. Whatever helps you relax, make sure you get at least one hour of calm every single day.

Physical fitness can also contribute to mood and make it easier for you to be self-motivated. Looking good also does wonders for our self-esteem. It makes you proud and adds to your confidence. You don't have to morph into a fitness freak overnight. Instead, start with small steps by creating a beginner's workout routine you can follow every day and later improve.

Taking on a new challenge allows you the opportunity to both fail and improve with. Before you begin the challenge, prepare mentally for both outcomes. Should things go wrong, use this opportunity to learn from the experience and come back better. If there are no issues, then know you have proven yourself to be capable. It is a direct challenge to your negative beliefs, and improves your self-esteem.

Building healthy self-esteem is a journey that is not completed all at once. So don't be disheartened if you wake up tomorrow feeling the same. Keep a journal to track your progress. This will make it easier for you to stay present in each choice, and celebrate your accomplishments in the future. Over time, you will find your new mindset has become a habit, and feel happier and healthier. Your elevated confidence will speak for itself, and you will find more people falling in line with your beliefs without question.

Chapter 2

Pointless Comparisons

"Comparison with myself brings improvement, comparison with others brings discontent." - Betty Jamie Chung

Have you ever found yourself comparing yourself to other people, whether it is a colleague, friend, family member, or celebrity? We often wonder if we are attractive, wealthy, or worthy enough of adoration. We find ourselves stuck in a thought loop, taking away from our motivation to do more. Negative thinking and comparisons lead to emotions like envy and jealousy. These emotions can lead to resentment of the people we compare ourselves to, and in the process sabotage those relationships.

Comparisons to other people are pointless, whether it is an upward or downward comparison. Upward comparisons can look like, "I wish I had a car like that," or "I wish I was that attractive." Whereas downward comparisons sound more like, "At least I have a job," or "I drive a nicer car than them."

Why Is It Pointless?

Comparing yourself to other people can steal valuable resources such as time and energy. At times, these comparisons may motivate you to make a change. In the end, you will find you spent all that time and energy trying to achieve goals set up for someone else. For example, imagine you just found out your colleague landed a high-paid promotion, and you envy them. So you start comparing yourself to them, wishing it was you instead. From the outside, this new position seems better than the one you currently have, not realizing all the new demands this position requires. It might demand more than you were willing to sacrifice, or the work could make you unhappy.

Downward comparisons are just as unhealthy, if not more. They create a sense of superiority within you. The aim is not to be better than everyone else. You don't want to be alone at the top of the mountain. Never look down on those who have less than you, especially if they are evidently struggling to survive. Use your higher status to be of service to them and help instead. It doesn't only have to be monetary help, but showing an act of kindness can go a long way.

The danger of comparisons is that it diminishes your sense of self-worth and stops you from finding your purpose in life. Before we look at how to stop comparing ourselves to others, I believe it is essential to understand why.

Perfection is an illusion. When we glance at someone and see them living an almost perfect life, we need to remind ourselves that these are the highlight reels. We never notice all that has come before and behind closed doors, including the late nights, the hard work, and the rejections.

In a competition, there are no friends, only rivals. Comparing yourself to others may lead to you being competitive by trying to accomplish what someone else already has, or more. It leads to jealousy within friendships and can make it hard to support your friends. When they accomplish their goals, you may find yourself pouting instead of clapping for them. Jealousy within friendships quickly causes deterioration, and over time you may find yourself with no genuine support in your corner.

You are who you are, why try to change that? Each person is unique and has special talents and quirks that nobody else has or can use the same way. By putting an end to comparison, you are freeing up valuable time that you can use towards finding out what those are. You only have control over one life, yours. Shift the focus back to yourself by investing all that time and energy to where it can make a difference.

There will always be someone who can do it better. In a world with over seven billion people, this is not unlikely. When you have a win-lose mindset, then this seems harsh. However, when you look at it from a healthy angle, you see nothing but the opportunity to learn and grow from the experience.

End the Comparisons Today

It can be hard to stop the comparisons as it is often happening subconsciously. It is not impossible, and if you follow the advice here, you can eventually train your mind to think differently. Remember, it is always possible to slip back into old habits. When this happens, all you need to do is remind yourself what you learned here. Have patience, but most importantly, be kind to yourself!
You might find yourself becoming envious or jealous of the person you so often compare your life or self to. The more you do this, the more room you make in your feelings for resentment. With this destructive behavior it is easier to sabotage healthy relationships and become even more isolated.
These habits may be hard to stop completely, but you can use this as an opportunity to transform negative thinking into a positive and healthy mindset. Below we look at ways to stop pointless comparisons and how to redirect this energy where it needs to be.

- Be aware.

Sometimes, we might not realize what is happening or exhibit this behavior unintentionally. By becoming aware of your thoughts and triggers, you can stop holding a negative mindset. A great way to identify your triggers is by writing them down or making a mental note when these feelings pop up. Keep a record of the times you have felt like less of a person because of someone else's influence and the situation you were in at the time. This will make it easier for you to avoid these triggers and mentally prepare when it happens again.

- Social media is a distorted version of real life.

Seeing posts from a friend or influence who just got engaged, went on a fancy vacation, bought a brand new sports car, or bought a home, remind yourself that these are highlight reels and not their everyday reality. Hard work, sacrifice, and late nights are what these images fail to show. Instead of wishing you were that person, use their experience to motivate yourself to work harder and strive towards your own goals.

- Focus on everything you have achieved so far.

Repeatedly focusing on other people can cause you to lose sight of yourself and how far you have already come. When you find yourself craving the success that your colleague seems blessed with, take that opportunity to remind yourself of everything you have accomplished in your life and how you got here. No matter the size or nature of the accomplishment, appreciate everything you are capable of doing.

- Find your joy.

Is the dream you are currently chasing yours? Have you sat down and thought about what you want from life? Is it something you want, or what someone else has? Questions like these can come in handy when evaluating what you put focus on. Take a moment to sit back, breathe, and write down all the things in life that currently make you happy. Next, write down your current goals. Compare the two lists and make sure you are not trying to achieve something that doesn't align with your happiness. Now create a new list of goals you want to accomplish for yourself. Break it down into smaller, manageable steps you can make each day. Remember, each journey begins with just one step in the right direction.

- The only person worth comparing yourself to is you.

The person you were yesterday, and the person you are now are two completely different people. Our everyday life and experiences continuously change us. We learn and grow. For example, you notice a pothole in the road while driving to work and make a mental note to avoid it in the future. That is a learning experience. Life is full of situations like this that we learn from, and we often take them for granted. When you feel sad about not reaching a goal, remind yourself of everything you have previously accomplished. Think of a situation that you handled well, the interview you rocked to get into your current position, or an assessment or exam you passed. Always strive to do better than yesterday. Try to learn something new every day. If you have routines, try to improve them by finding smarter ways to do them. Read a book, even if you start with just one page a day.

- Practice gratitude.

Gratitude teaches us to appreciate everything you have - a roof over your head, a warm meal to eat, work to put effort into. Whatever it is, find new ways to be grateful. Think about the people in your life and how lucky you are to have unlimited support and love. Being thankful will teach you to look at yourself with a healthier mindset. It improves self-love and the feelings you have for other people. Gratitude eventually leads to contentment.

Even with practice, you may still find negative emotions like jealousy or envy creeping in. These emotions do nothing but cause unhappiness and allow resentment to build. However, it is possible to repurpose these emotions into something positive, like motivation. Follow these simple steps to start leading a healthier life now!

1. Identify the cause. Why are you jealous? Are you jealous because your friend got a well-paying job? If you are, would you pursue the same field? Are you envious of the fact that they seem happier than you? Are you just frustrated by your job and wish you could have another? Identify the root cause of your emotions. Use this as a starting point to turning your life around.

2. Know you can do it. Understand that you are more than capable of achieving your goals. Believe in yourself. Instead of being envious, use this as an opportunity to learn more. If you are jealous of a colleague, use this opportunity to talk to them and find out more about them, and more about how they got where they are. Ask for tips and advice that can help you get to a better position. Do your research and create everyday tasks that can help you to reach your goals.

3. Celebrate your success. Celebrating yourself gives you the motivation you need to keep striving forward. Acknowledging your achievements, significant or otherwise, allows you the opportunity to capitalize and improve at the same time. For example, if you woke up this morning and completed all your chores, celebrate that! Make it a goal to do this every day, then add to it. Add a goal that will improve wellness, like meditation or a fun way to exercise.

4. Work on you. Take a walk, drink water, calm your mind, play a game, or read a book. The things you can do to improve yourself are endless. Make it a goal to do at least one thing every day. Start small, and then move your way forward from there. So, if you took a five-minute walk today, aim for six-minutes next time. The increase might seem insignificant at first, but if you follow this routine long-term, you will gradually notice an improvement.

Changing the way you think can improve your life. Thinking with a negative mindset can paralyze you, making it harder for you to reach the goals you set for yourself. In the next chapter, we look into mindsets and how a positive one can change your life!

Chapter 3

Abundance vs Scarcity

"When you want something, all the universe conspires in helping you achieve it." - Paulo Coelho

Most people live within a scarcity mindset. They might think of a few things with an abundance mindset, but overall their view is limited. This type of thought process can negatively affect your life. In this chapter, we look at what these mindsets mean. We will also look at ways to transition into a more positive way of life.

Scarcity Mindset

Have you ever felt like there is not enough in the world? Do you often view things like relationships, job opportunities, and time as limited? These are signs of having a scarcity mindset. Having a scarcity mindset means that you see the world as finite. In many areas of life, it can cause you to think there will never be enough. For example, we sometimes cling to relationships because we believe no one else will love us (like this) again. We stick to a career path because it is all we know. We do less with our time because we are afraid to waste it on uncertainty.

To an extent, having this type of mindset can help you. It's a short-term idea that can have long-term consequences. Thinking this way can cause a sense of urgency in your life. The issue is we focus only on immediate needs, and lose sight of the long run. Let's take a closer look at what this can mean.

A long time ago, I had a scarcity mindset, particularly in relationships. I had been in a toxic relationship with someone for five years. Although I knew the relationship was not good for me, I found it hard to leave them because of my thought process. I had become clingy, needy, and couldn't rationalize walking away because I thought I would never get another chance at love. Having a scarcity mindset during this time meant I felt love and security in a relationship for a short length of time at the cost of my mental health in the long run. Admittedly, we can develop this mindset from society. Movies often portray love to be rare, and we only have one soulmate. At school, we receive trophies and medals for being a top achiever, further fueling the idea of competition and rivalry. Friends and family will often question our plans for the future, making it seem as though true happiness only lies in respectable professions with a high paycheck. Many of us don't realize it, but this way of thinking can be dangerous. It limits the scope of possibilities and can prevent you from finding where your passion truly lies.

There are five ways a scarcity mindset affects you:

- Time is running out. The fear of not having enough time can often paralyze you. Meaning, you may sometimes find yourself thinking about how little time you have left without actually doing anything at the moment. You may start to obsess about things like finding the right job or partner out of fear for the future. You may sometimes feel hopeless and begin to throw away your goals and dreams out of a fear of being too old to accomplish them.

- Negative thought patterns. A scarcity mindset limits you to think pessimistically. You tend to focus on the negatives and what could go wrong. You forget to think about the good and what could go right. You often talk yourself out of opportunities before you even try. You live in fear of the unknown. It becomes difficult for you to leave unhealthy situations, negatively impacting your mental or physical health. You also miss out on a lot of opportunities, decreasing your chances of finding happiness.

- Fear of missing out. This can manifest in many different ways. In relationships, it can manifest as clinginess. We refuse to leave unhealthy situations because we fear that we will never have another partner. Many people are afraid of being alone or being single. They would rather stay in those relationships than risk missing out on love or physical affection. We stay in careers that make us unhappy because we fear the loss of income and financial security. This fear can also manifest a need to compete. When you think everything is limited, it makes you want to win so that you don't miss out on the reward.

- Greed and overindulgence. This is a side effect of a scarcity mindset. We feel the need to obtain our wants and needs immediately because we see time and money as limited resources. Those with a mindset of scarcity tend to become addicted to the feeling instant gratification provides. That usually leads to compulsive and excessive spending and overeating.

- It will never be enough. The problem with being afraid of the future is that you tend to sacrifice today's happiness to enjoy more of it tomorrow. Unfortunately, tomorrow never comes because you never have enough. There will always be something new that you see and want. It prevents you from noticing all that you already have and achieved, even if it is a lot. It also prevents you from being grateful and celebrating yourself.

Abundance Mindset

An abundance mindset is the polar opposite of a scarcity mindset, and offers you long-term benefits. When you think with abundance, you view life as unlimited. You understand that there are more than enough resources for everyone to share and still have leftovers. You also understand that there is sufficient time to live a meaningful and happy life. You always think of the glass as half full and refillable. Looking at life with abundance means that you can see life as a journey with obstacles that you can overcome. You are not afraid of the future, and for that reason, you can plan better and make wiser decisions.

This mindset helps to abolish your fears, like the fear of missing out. It allows you the freedom to take calculated risks, increasing your chance of a range of opportunities. You are less likely to stay in situations that make you uncomfortable or unhappy, improving your mental health in the long run. You're also less likely to feel threatened by competition, seeing it as a learning curve instead. While people with a scarcity mindset compete with each other for the top, people with an abundance mindset will work together and share it. They also tend to cheer people on instead of putting them down or insulting them. They genuinely want other people to succeed.

People with this type of mindset are usually givers. Even if they don't have much themselves, they still give. It stems from the fact that they don't see resources as limited in any way. We believe that the more we give, the more we get. They are not attached to things like money or knowledge, as they believe there is always more.

People who think with a scarcity mindset are usually alone and aim to win. When you think abundantly, you begin to value working with other people and sharing your knowledge. You aren't afraid of anyone stealing your success because you understand that it is an unlimited resource. Below, we look at common traits shared by people with an abundance mindset.

- Always have the bigger picture in mind. The unlimited world provides benefits, like being able to think outside the box. You get more creative when setting goals for yourself and think with a clearer mind. Your mind is not foggy with fear.

- Unlimited potential. When you understand that there are enough resources for everyone, you also realize that the potential to do more is endless. You do not limit yourself and take more chances. You also believe in yourself.

- Happiness. Viewing the world with an unlimited mindset leads to overall happiness and contentment. It is because no matter whose turn it is to succeed today, whether it's your promotion or a colleague's promotion, it makes you happy. You can genuinely support your friends because your need to compete no longer exists.

- Change. We embrace change because we understand that it leads to more opportunities and success. People with a limited view of life tend to be more fearful of change, preventing themselves from new experiences. It is a valuable learning curve, for there is no better teacher than experience.

- Appreciation. When you have a healthy, unlimited mindset, you can be grateful for everything you already have. It also allows you to see how lucky you are to have everything that you own and prompts the need to give to the less fortunate. The act of giving, be it time or money, increases your happiness in life.

How to Change Your Mindset

After spending a lifetime within the reaches or boundaries of a scarcity mindset, it can be harder to transition to a healthier, abundance mindset. The transition can be long, and you may sometimes find yourself regressing into old habits. Try not to be hard on yourself when this happens. Remember, there is more than enough time! After relapsing, you need to revisit these techniques and implement them again. Over time, it will become your natural way of life. Let us take a look at five easy steps to a healthier mindset:

1. Look around yourself. Take note of everything that you have, all the goals you have already accomplished. Always try to focus on the bright side of situations. Remind yourself why you are worthy of everything you desire. Remember the hard work and passion you have put into getting yourself to this point, and remind yourself of everything you are still capable of accomplishing. By doing this, you make it easier for you to celebrate yourself. You make it easier to love

and be proud of yourself, and this builds healthy self-confidence.

2. Hangout with the like-minded. Always surround yourself with people who think the way you do or strive to be like. Surrounding yourself with negative people will rub off on you, depriving you of opportunity and success. When you surround yourself with those who think with abundance, you are guaranteed support and success. When people with a limited mindset stop you from taking risks, the unlimited thinkers are sure to support and cheer you on.

3. Support others without expecting anything in return. You can support others by lending a non-judgmental ear when they are having problems, teaching them something from your experience, or cheering for their success. This energy exchange is sure to cement long-term, healthy relationships. It also helps you develop a win-win mentality, leading to situations where everyone gets something of value, and nobody has to lose. A mindset like this allows you to work better with other people. Friendlier people are also able to

network better, increasing their chance for future opportunities.

4. Practice gratitude. Studies have shown that this behavior leads to improved physical and mental well-being. It breeds contentment in life. When you focus on everything you already have, it makes it harder for you to want more. It is important to be grateful for everything, including the air you breathe, the shoes on your feet, and the comfort your bed provides every night. A great way to incorporate gratitude into your daily life is to write down at least three things you are grateful for each day. You can do this in the morning after you wake up to create a healthy mindset for the rest of your day or in the evening before you go to sleep. This clears your mind and makes it easier for you to rest.

5. Create opportunities. Train yourself to see everything available to you, unlimited opportunities and resources. When we focus too intently, it's easy to lose sight of what's in front of us. Train your mind to loosen its focus. Think of everything as possible and you will experience more. A simple question

you can ask, "If I could be anything I wanted right now, what would it be?" The answer to this question can open up desire in this moment and spur creative thinking. Use this answer to frame new goals for yourself and open the road to unlimited opportunities.

Always remember, our thoughts shape our reality. Having the right mindset gives you a better chance to feel happy. When we are happy, we develop a zest for life. It makes us want to set high goals and achieve them. We lose our inhibitions and leave our comfort zones, taking more risks and achieving more than we would have had we been feeling depressed. Repeat the ten abundance mindset affirmations to yourself each day to make the transition easier:

1. I believe in myself and my potential.

2. I am worthy.

3. I am capable of success.

4. I am grateful for all that I have.

5. I am brave and confident.

6. I am proud of myself.

7. I have the money I need.

8. I deserve to love and be loved.

9. I love my body.

10. I believe there is enough for everyone.

Chapter 4

Appreciate Reality

"We suffer more often in imagination than in reality."
-Seneca

We regularly dwell on things we don't have. We spend our days looking at fancy houses, expensive cars, and the latest technology. It's easy to lose time admiring our favorite celebrity's lives. We wish, with all of our hearts, to have what they have. It often puts us in a bad mood and can quickly depreciate our mental health. It leaves us feeling unsatisfied and unfulfilled. In the end, we believe that we are a failure for not having what they have. By the end of this chapter, you should be able to think of yourself with pride, and not judge yourself based on what you think you lack. A measure of success is not based on others, it is based on you.

When was the last time you took a moment to pause and look around? Have you ever stopped to appreciate life? We are so caught up in chasing our dreams that we forget to appreciate everything we have already achieved. It prevents you from noticing all your past successes, and you fail to reward yourself. Doing this deprives you of the celebration you crave. When you feel like you haven't accomplished much in life, it can cause you to grow resentment for yourself and those you admire. You can feel this way for a multitude of reasons. However, the most common one would be because we simply do not praise ourselves enough. We forget to remind ourselves of how proud we are for making it this far.

When you stop to appreciate reality, it does more than open your eyes to how lucky you are. Research has shown that being grateful and appreciative can also have health benefits such as lowered depression, lower blood pressure, and increased dopamine and serotonin in the body.

Ways to Stay Grounded

It can be easy to lose track of your accomplishments and possessions while chasing your dreams. We tend to focus on the destination and forget to enjoy the journey. To help you lead a life of gratitude and appreciation, I have designed a few techniques that you can attempt every day.

Keep a jar of blessings. Each morning or evening, write a small note on what you are grateful for today and place it in a designated jar. Whenever you feel depressed or find yourself wanting more, read your notes to remind yourself of everything you already have and appreciate. It is a great way to get a quick boost of happiness and confidence.

Reduce screen and social media use especially if you tend to become transfixed on other people's lives. Research has shown that social media is closely associated with depression negative moods. Experts suggest using social media for no more than 20 minutes a day. Spending too much time here means that you are not spending enough time in reality where you have control and make a difference.

Do your research on the disadvantaged and underprivileged - Educating yourself on the less fortunate comes with many advantages. An awareness of those who are less privileged than you helps to cultivate appreciation and gratitude for the life you have. Research has also shown that the act of giving prompts our bodies to release oxytocin, allowing us to live a happier and more fulfilling life. Volunteer at a local shelter and speak to them yourself. Always speak to them with kindness and respect, as you would any other person. This breeds humility and compassion within you. At the same time, witnessing the struggles of the world breeds compassion and humility. It allows you to cherish everything you own and have accomplished. You can take it one step further by offering help where it's needed, but this should be your choice.

Write down memories. Keep a journal in which you record your fondest memories. Every day, write down at least one thing that made you happy. These can be things you did alone or with people you love. This method keeps positivity within arms reach when you need a pick-me-up. Remind yourself of what makes you happy, and then go out and make more memories!

Create daily, positive affirmations. Before you get out of bed each morning, make it a habit to repeat kind words to yourself. You can create a mantra. A mantra is a phrase that you can repeat to yourself at any time. You can make up your own mantra, or search the internet for an existing one. There are different mantras used for different purposes. Tell yourself that you are worthy, and you are loved. Some common affirmations you can use are, "I believe in myself," "I am proud of who I am," and "I am not perfect, and that is okay."

Have a self-care day at least once every month. On this day, the only person who should matter is you. Make yourself a priority and indulge. You don't have to go out and splurge on expensive items, sometimes all you need is a hot bath and some time alone to unwind. Tap into your needs and appreciate yourself!

Celebrate the little things. We always celebrate big moments, like birthdays or anniversaries. Very rarely do we appreciate the little achievements in life. An example of something we can celebrate is crossing something off our to-do list like cleaning a room or doing the laundry. Reward yourself by doing something you enjoy and reminding yourself of how proud you are. Other little things to be proud of each day are:

- Good health. Even if you are not in the greatest shape, remember it could be worse.

- A roof over your head. Most people take this for granted. So remind yourself how tough life would be if you were homeless.
- Breath. You wouldn't be here without it.
- The ability to see and comprehend.
- Nature. Not only is it beautiful, but it provides us with oxygen and food.
- Friends and family. Having supportive people in your corner is always something to be grateful for.

There are an infinite amount of things that we take for granted in life. All of which deserve appreciation.

Be Present

Living in the 'now' means that you are aware of everything that is happening around you. You are not lost in your mind, thinking about the past and the future. It is the key to happiness. Recent studies have also shown mindfulness to have a positive impact on your mental health. It reduces stress, anxiety, and depression. That is not to say that we should stop thinking about our past and future - we should think of them in small doses but with a purpose. We think of the past to remember a good memory or to remind ourselves of how far we have come. We think of the future to set goals and a direction for our lives. Having these thoughts is important, but we should not allow them to consume our lives. Read further to find out how you can start living in the present moment.

Calm your mind, take a deep breath. Calming your mind clears it from confusion and worry. It allows you to see more clearly with a logical mind. You will also be able to make better decisions, drastically improving the quality of your life. Don't focus on problems. Instead, focus on solutions. In the following chapter, we dive into problem-solving and the best way to identify and solve issues efficiently.

Mindfulness Meditation

Religions and spiritual faiths have preached the benefits of meditation for centuries. In recent years, studies have shown the effectiveness of this practice. Meditation brings the mind back to the now, allowing you to embrace living in the present. It can also benefit you in other ways, like reducing stress, tension, and body aches.

You can take your exercises one step further with meditation. There are many different ways, so you can take your time trying and choosing the best one for your lifestyle. With enough practice you can even put together your own form of meditation if the traditional methods don't work for you.

A sitting meditation usually involves sitting legs crossed with your eyes closed, keeping your back in an upright posture. With this meditation, your thoughts should focus on your breath. Use deep breathing exercises, and clear your mind of everything but what is happening in this moment. Focus on how you feel, and visualize the benefits this breathing is providing. It is normal for a beginner's mind to wander, so when it does, take note of the reason and return your focus to your breath. You can practice for ten minutes each day. Choose a place that is comfortable with minimal distraction.

If you are the kind of person who finds it difficult to sit still for too long, try a walking or moving meditation. Walking meditation is fairly simple. It involves you pacing in a large, open space; it can be a room, at a park or at the beach. Your hands stay at your sides, or you can clasp them behind your back. Your eyes should stay open with any movement for safety, of course. As with all forms of meditation, your back should always stay in an upright position. Focus on your breathing, but also be aware of the activity happening around you. The great thing about this meditation is that it can be attempted any time and anywhere. You can practice at work when you're walking from your office to the meeting room, or at home from your bedroom to the kitchen. Try and practice it as often as you can, at least ten minutes each day to really see a difference.

Moving meditation is a bit complex in that it requires a specific set of movements. There are many ways to practice this sort of meditation. Some common examples can include tai chi, yoga, and pilates. If you are not familiar with any of these practices, I suggest searching for the many videos available on YouTube to get a better idea of these movements. You can also join groups online that share these interests, or find a local class. This form of meditation provides more than just benefits for the mind. It also helps to keep you fit and active, acting as a natural self-confidence boost.

Change your perspective about life. Your opinion is the only one that matters. View life as a blessing rather than a burden, and witness the boost of happiness and gratitude you will experience. Reality is everything in front of you at this moment. It is not the past, and it is not the future. Those are just concepts. Remind yourself of this fact every day. Your future success is dependent on the choices that you make today. So take a deep breath, and start appreciating your reality right now!

Chapter 5

Self-Motivation and Your Goals

"If you want to be happy, set a goal that commands your thoughts, liberates your energy and inspires your hopes."
- Andrew Carnegie

In the first grade, our teacher had a question for the class. "What do you want to be when you grow up?" She walked around the class listening to the hopeful responses of my bright-eyed classmates. Some wanted to be doctors, while others wanted to be astronauts or lawyers. I couldn't help but feel embarrassed because I had no idea what I wanted to be. So I listened to the different answers and picked the most common one, a teacher.

That is the story of how I went through my education, providing the same half-hearted answer to anyone who would ask, all because I did not know what I wanted out of life. As I got older it morphed into "What are you studying?" or "What is your degree in?"; I learned more about the profession and what it would entail if I took this choice seriously. It was only after years of letting everyone think I knew what my dream job was, did I realize just how much I hated the idea. How many of us still do this? How many of us are living lives based on someone else's vision? Are you currently pursuing goals that genuinely make you happy, or are you just following a dream that was never yours?

In this chapter, we aim to uncover where our happiness lies. When we create goals based on our vision and ideas, it becomes easier to reach those goals. It makes us happy and a willing participant in our own lives. Set goals that align with your happiness as well as values. We work harder when we know we will enjoy the outcome. When there is a tinge of unhappiness associated with our goals, we tend to want to give up. If an obstacle arises, we don't work as hard to overcome them. If we fail, we shutdown instead of learning from our mistakes and trying again. Most of us are not even aware of our unhappiness until it's too late. By then, we don't bother to create new goals because of our fear of failure. So before we can learn how to set appropriate goals, let us first find ourselves and discover our happiness.

Listed below are five questions you can ask yourself. Try to complete this exercise at the end of every week, and you will eventually be able to give yourself genuine answers after much soul-searching. Please note, this will take courage to complete and there are no right or wrong answers. Feel free to write them out on your own, answer now, come back later and add more. Whatever process works best for you is the right one. For best results, review the first three chapters before attempting this section.

If there was no such thing as failure, what would you want to be? Most of us allow fear to lead our lives. We base our goals, hopes, and dreams on how likely it is to achieve these things. We rarely create goals that seem unlikely or too good to be true. We want to live in that mansion with cool cars and fancy clothes like our favorite celebrity, but we don't aim for that because we know that it is unlikely to happen or that we will ever be famous. So, if there was no such thing as failure and everyone is on a level playing field, anything is possible, what would you be doing right now? What choices would you make and how are they different to the real ones today?

Who are you? One of the most commonly asked questions. Interviews, social media bios, dating profiles, or when you meet someone for the first time. As common as this question is, it is mostly answered in an aloof, broad manner. If you had to deliver a two-minute speech on who you are as a person, what you want out of life, and what matters to you, what would that speech sound like? Write it out, ask a loved one to listen if you feel brave. Now try answering this question based on the many different scenarios like in an interview, or on a first date.

Where does your moral compass point? Your moral compass is what sets the general direction of your life. Your moral compass comprises things you find valuable and hold close to your heart. These can include family values, supportive friendships, living with integrity, and showing kindness. These values guide the way we make decisions. They can also help in setting up goals that don't conflict with who you are.

Where does your happiness lie? This one relates to your moral compass, so only answer it once you have completed question three. Consider the dreams you have. Ask yourself if it will make you happy now that you know what your core values are. For example, if a family is one of your core values, would taking a job that requires most of your time make you genuinely happy?

If money was not an issue, what would you be doing? Most people tend to create goals with money in mind. We are always worried about our financial status because we need money to survive. So, if the need for money was non-existent, what would you be doing with your time? Try to think outside the box with this one. The possibilities are limitless. These things may not be possible, but you will begin to develop goals that can get you as close as possible. You will also have a better understanding of what makes you happy in life.

How to Set Goals

Before we can set our goals, we first need to understand what they are. Many people find it arduous to pursue their goals because they fail to distinguish them from what is supposed to be self-improvement habits. So, do you find yourself setting the same goals every year? Do you wake every morning, claiming to get something done but don't? Don't worry, you're not alone in this.

In January many people set a 'goal' to exercise every day. After the first few weeks or days, they give up and have the same resolution next year. The issue with this is, exercise is not a goal. It is a self-improvement habit.

To create a goal out of it, you need to figure out why you are exercising. Whether it is to lose weight or maybe you are training to compete in a marathon. Maybe you just want to be in better shape and eat healthy. These are goals. They make it easier for you to accomplish because you have steps to take, and a destination in mind. Just "exercising every day" has no destination or obvious step, this makes it easier for you to get off track and go back to old patterns.

To achieve your goals, you need to have a destination in mind and a willingness to get there. That is why you must create goals that will make you happy. Use this step-by-step method to create and achieve more detailed goals.

1. Visualize what you want to achieve. Picture what the result should look like and all the work required to get there. If you have many goals, think about the most important ones first. Now ask yourself, is this something that would make you happy in the long run? Is this worth the time and energy needed to accomplish it? Are you willing to do everything it takes to achieve it? If you answer 'no' to any of these questions, this goal might not be as important as you think, and there is a possibility that this is not what you truly desire.

2.   Be specific. Now that you have a goal in mind, it's time to narrow it down. It can be easy to lose focus on the destination when you have no clear direction to travel. So let's say your goal is to lose weight. This goal has no specifics. How much weight do you want to lose? When do you want to lose weight? Is the amount of weight you want to lose realistic and healthy? Look into the tools you need to refine your goal. Morph the wording to be more like, "I want to lose 10 pounds by [insert date]." Now you have a deadline and a target so you can make a better fitness plan.

3.   Write it down. Now that you know what you want out of life, it's time to set it in stone. Write down your goals. Make sure the most important goal is right at the top. It will be your priority. Writing out your goals means you are turning an idea into a plan. Keep your goals where you can see them, stick them on the fridge or your mirror. It will work as a daily reminder to work hard and strive for what you want.

4.   Plan it out. Remember, failing to plan is planning to fail. When you don't have a plan, it means that you don't know how to achieve

it, only that you want to achieve it. With this step, I suggest getting creative. Use color, and write in large, bold fonts. Not only does this cement a plan in your mind, but it will make you excited every single time you look at it. We want our journey to be fun, not a chore. Do some research to understand what is required to reach your goal. Then, write out a step-by-step action plan.

5. Give yourself a deadline. By giving yourself a deadline, you create a sense of urgency within. Make sure that each step in your plan has a complete-by-date. Include milestones, and create a reward system. Only reward yourself if you have reached a milestone on time. It motivates you to work harder and stick to your schedule.

6. Ready? Set. Go! Now that you know what you want and how to get there, it is time to begin your journey. Try to put your plan in action as soon as you can. The longer you wait, the more you procrastinate. Always remember these wise words, "Procrastination is the enemy of success."

7. Evaluate yourself. At the end of every week, sit down to evaluate your progress. Not only does this remind you of how far you have already come, but it also reminds you of how close to the finish line you are. It serves as motivation to keep pushing through to the end. If need be, you can also use this time to reevaluate your steps and make necessary adjustments.

Self-Motivation

Sticking to your new plan of action can be tough, so here are some expert techniques to help you stay on track.

- Always believe in yourself! Because if you don't, you'll lack the confidence needed to reach your end goal.

- Never give up! Especially on the hard days. Keep pushing; keep moving forward. If you fail, learn from the experience and try again. Always be willing to have your own back, and pick yourself up.

- Never stop learning! Knowledge is infinite, and you can never have enough. An informed person is always able to make the best choices. So keep yourself informed, especially on your goals.

- If you start something, finish it! Completing tasks makes you happier. Research has shown that our brains release small amounts of the feel good hormone, dopamine every time we complete a task or experience success. Use this as motivation to finish what you have started.

- Take care of yourself! Remember, your well-being should always be your top priority. If your mental and physical health is not up to par, it can be difficult and even dangerous to attempt to reach your goals. Drink enough water, eat clean, and make sure you get enough restful sleep. It will make you more efficient in completing tasks. You also feel better, meaning you are more enthusiastic and motivated to reach your goals.

Remember, one step at a time. Do not overburden yourself, as you can quickly become demotivated, unhappy, and unhealthy. Self-motivation does not come naturally, so it is up to us to practice techniques to help us. Always keep in mind that doing nothing guarantees 100% failure, so always aim to do something, no matter how insignificant you think it is. In the next chapter, we take a closer look at how we can effectively deal with failure and why failing can contribute to your success. We will also learn about criticism, why it is healthy, and how to effectively deal with it.

Chapter 6

Failure

"Failure is simply the opportunity to begin again, this time more intelligently." - Henry Ford

Failure is crucial to success. Did you know that Thomas Edison, the man who created the lightbulb, failed 1000 times before he succeeded? Publishers rejected J.K. Rowling 12 times before giving her a chance. Walt Disney's superiors fired him because they thought he lacked imagination. The list of household names who first failed before experiencing endless success goes on. But do you know what they all have in common? The will to never give. They never stopped trying, even when success seemed impossible. They gained the admiration and respect of billions of people across the world.

When Edison was asked how it felt to fail 1000 times, he responded by saying he did not fail 1000 times, he just found 1000 ways that didn't work. That is the answer of someone with the will to never give up. If Edison overcame more than the average amount of obstacles, what is stopping you from overcoming yours? The likely answer is fear. We fear failure, but the problem is we are looking at it from the wrong perspective. We still view them as failures, when we should be viewing them as learning curves. In this chapter, we will change the way we view our failure. In doing so, we can eradicate fear, making it easy to keep pushing forward.

It is important to understand that failure does not mean that you are not good enough, it just means that you need to approach the situation differently. It can teach you so much about life and yourself. Failure helps to keep us grounded and gives us the experience we need to navigate a world that can be cruel. Failure is not a dead-end. It is one step closer to success. When you fail at something, it doesn't mean that you have achieved nothing. It means you have now learned of at least one way your idea will not work.

Why Failure Is Important

Failure helps to build character and strength. If you had to succeed immediately in everything in life, chances are you wouldn't appreciate it as much. When we fail and come back from it, we allow ourselves to cherish the success that follows.
It also eradicates fear. Most often than not, we don't attempt to reach our goals because of a fear of failure. The more you try, the more chance there will be to fail. It is not a bad thing, because the more you fail, the more accustomed you become. Being accustomed and welcoming of failure eradicates that fear. Without fear, you begin to allow yourself to try new things, create higher goals, and get out of your comfort zone.
View failure as an opportunity to become more resilient at facing odds. If you fail 99 times, make sure you try 100 times. Whatever you do, never stop trying!

How to Use Failure to Your Advantage

The most common mistake we make when trying to reach our goals is focusing on the wrong thing. We tend to focus on not failing rather than seeing the results. What sets you apart from a true failure is the actions you take in the face of adversity. Below, we look at the proper steps to take after a mishap.

- Take accountability - This is the most important as it can be the deciding factor in whether your peers see you as just somebody or a leader. A leader is someone who is always accountable for the actions he or she takes. If you make a mistake, admit it. Do not stay quiet, and do not try to blame anyone else. Doing so also helps to build character and courage, attributes required to reach your goals.

- Explain, not excuse - If there is a reason, feel free to mention it. Do not make an excuse. For example, if you miss an opportunity because of a deadline, say, "I missed the opportunity because I missed the deadline." Making an excuse would sound like, "I missed the deadline because she didn't tell me, it's not my fault."

- Fix your mistake - Owning up to your mistake is only the first step; the real test comes after. This part is crucial and requires emotional intelligence. If you fail, make sure to come up with a plan to fix it. Communicate with all parties involved about what your intentions are. Never wait for someone else to clean up after you, and always be accountable for your actions.

- Don't make the same mistake twice - Once you have owned up to your mistake and resolved it, make a note. Remember what happened, what went wrong, and how you can prevent the same mistake from happening in the future. The true measure of success is the ability to learn from your mistakes.

- Don't give up - As soon as you fail, get back up, re-evaluate, and try again. Waiting allows you the opportunity to convince yourself to give up. If you don't try again, you allow your fear back in to stop you from succeeding.

- Change your perspective, change your life - The way you deal with mistakes is determined by how you view them. We tend to blame ourselves for mistakes. What you can do instead is look at the situation from a different side. Remind yourself that this situation occurred because of an action you took, rather than a personal trait. We can control our actions, but we can't control who we are. Blaming a personality trait reinforces the idea that we had no control over the situation, stopping us from continuing. Admitting our actions allows us the opportunity to change them and move forward.

- Be optimistic - Always stay hopeful about the future. Remind yourself that this will not last forever. When we talk about Henry Ford, we never mention his failures. We only talk about all he achieved as the result of his hard work. Always keep in mind that failure is a possibility, but you have the tools to overcome it.

Problem Solving
Learning to deal with failure is just the first step. The next step is learning how to solve the problem to move past it. At times, it might not be obvious as to where we went wrong, making it difficult to avoid the same mistake in the future.
Use the following method to identify the problem:
1. Write down the process you followed as accurately as you can recall.
2. Try to identify where the problem occurred (ask for help or do the research).

3. If possible, repeat the process to identify the
    problem.

Now you can move on to the next step, solving the
problem. Create multiple solutions, as this allows
you to prepare for possible failure, but it also allows
you a higher chance of success. Get creative with
your solutions, and make sure they are actionable.
You can create them by modifying your original
process or creating a new one. I suggest having a
variety of both, especially if you are finding it
difficult to identify the problem. Next, rearrange
your list of solutions so that the one with the most
potential to succeed is at the top. Eliminate
solutions that might not succeed or have a low
chance. It will ensure a refined list.
Once you have identified the best possible solution,
it is time to put it into action. It's best to do this as
soon as you can so you can avoid talking yourself
out of trying. Once your plan is in motion, it is
essential to monitor its progress. You should be able
to solve problems as soon as they arise or prevent
possible errors. On completion of your plan,
evaluate the success. If it has still failed, move on to
your next possible solution. If your plan is a success,
determine if this solution will work with similar
problems in the future. If you find that it will not
work later on, you may want to go back to the
drawing board and take further action.

Your problem-solving skills can be the deciding factor in whether you achieve or not. In order to solve issues quickly and effectively, you need to hone your analytical, creative, and logical skills. Find activities you can do daily to keep these skills sharp, and always be ready to solve a problem. Keep in mind, when you fail, there will be people who will be ready to criticize you. Next, let's take a look at how to acknowledge and deal with criticism.

Dealing With Criticism

We can't control what people say to us, but we can control how we choose to respond to them. Criticism comes in many forms, usually unsolicited, and can sometimes be harsh. However, there is an upside to the benefits it provides us if you deal with it correctly.

The first benefit is personal growth. In many ways, it can help you to see things from different perspectives. It helps to expand your thinking, allowing you to come up with ideas you might not have considered before. It's not always easy to take an honest look at yourself and acknowledge your flaws, but you can't grow if you don't fix them.

The second benefit is that it nurtures your emotional intelligence. It teaches you humility and how to control your feelings. By learning to accept criticism, you teach yourself to not respond based on how you feel. It can also help to uncover unresolved trauma, especially when the criticism is harsh. It also allows you to choose peace over conflict, so remember to make the right choice!

Criticism also helps to boost your self-confidence. Being on the receiving end of harsh judgment can often bring out your insecurities. Seize the opportunity to work on and heal from them. When you rid yourself of insecurities, you realize that having flaws is normal, we all have them, even the perfect celebrity. Learn to accept them, and witness your self-confidence soar.

Listen to understand, not respond. Listen to the feedback assuming that the person is trying to help you, and not harm you. Listen with an open mind and wait for them to finish what they are saying. Never jump to conclusions, as this can deter you from understanding the critic. When your critic has finished speaking, repeat key points to make sure you have understood. Thank the person for their input to show that you are appreciative of the help they offered.

Stay calm, relax your body, and keep your arms unfolded. Practice deep breathing so that you can relieve stress and tension from your body. Doing so allows you to be more receptive and accepting. It also relieves the need to lash out and create a scene. Don't be afraid to ask questions. Get clarity on things you don't understand or don't agree with. Be willing to have an honest, respectful conversation. You should also ask for advice on how to improve, this will help you to create new solutions from a fresh perspective. Getting a second opinion will help you to discern whether the critic was accurate, and also gain more ideas from a third perspective.

Use the criticism received to improve yourself. Embrace it, and never allow yourself to view it as an attack on who you are, rather, use it as a learning curve. Also remember, you are human. It is natural to feel emotional or defensive but never allow your emotions to control you. Remind yourself that this feedback does not define who you are, and you are not a failure.

Conclusion

Before we conclude, I would like you to ponder upon this quote by Mandy Hale, "Happiness is letting go of what you think your life is supposed to look like and celebrating it for everything that it is." I love this quote because of the truth behind it. When you stop wishing for more and simply enjoy what you already have, you will attain true happiness.

By now, you should possess the skills needed to reach your goals no matter what happens. The key is to keep trying. Reach for your happiness before attempting to reach for your other goals. By doing this, you are already cultivating the motivation needed to push forward. You are giving yourself the strength needed to fearlessly face adversity head-on.

Practice the techniques mentioned here every day. It is important to practice them on good days, and bad. Never stop working on yourself, even once you have reached your goals. The only thing constant in your life is you. So give yourself the most kindness, respect, and love you have to offer. Treat yourself as you would treat your closest friend, and never let yourself down. Always have your own back. Cultivate a willingness within to pick yourself up when you fall, dust yourself off, and move forward.

Always remember that you are unique, and there is no one else out there like you. It is unfair to compare yourself to other people, as their life is completely different to yours. We are shaped by the choices we make in life, so unless someone else has made the exact same choices and has the exact same experiences as you, which is highly unlikely, there is no need to compare yourself to them. The only person you can compare yourself to is who you were yesterday, as you know what they have been through.

Do not rush yourself to complete your goals based on someone else's timeline. You are you, and you work at your own pace. Create your goals with this in mind. If you notice that another person has what you are aiming for, remind yourself that if they can do it, so can you. Stay away from negative emotions like envy and jealousy. These emotions can quickly lead to unhappiness and prompt you to do the wrong things.

Instead, change your perspective. Look at them as a goal rather than a competition. Try to befriend this person, you can gain valuable insight on how to get what you want. Who knows, you might even gain a valuable and supportive friend. Chances this is what you are aiming for. True intelligence is knowing when to seize an opportunity. Do not sabotage yourself by burning bridges out of jealousy. In the end, it's not worth it if you're all alone at the top. It's lonely, so make sure you take as many people with you as possible.

I can't stress enough the importance of starting a journal. You will not regret it. In this journal, I want you to write down all of your aspirations in life. Even if they seem silly, write it down. You can also include things like your random thoughts, something that made you smile, dreams and hopes, as well as your memories. Make this journal creative, and pour your soul into it. Make sure to update every day so you can keep track of your progress and growth. At the end of every month, go through this journal so that you can see what has changed. Has any of your morals or dreams changed? If so, be sure to adjust your goals accordingly.

Remember to look at life with an unlimited mindset. Let go of your fear that there isn't enough time or resources for everyone. The world has more than enough resources for everyone to get what they want and still have more leftover. Rid yourself of the idea that everything has to be a competition or that we are in a race to see who can get the most out of life. We are on this Earth to contribute, not to keep taking without ever giving something back. After all, we are nothing but passing visitors, and the world will still be here long after we leave.

Learn to be compassionate and humble. Treat everyone you meet with the same kindness and respect that you would expect for yourself. If you are in a position to try and help those who are less fortunate than you. Not only will it remind you of why you need to be grateful for everything you have, but it will also help you to create bonds and strengthen your community.

Whenever you feel like a failure, remind yourself of everything you have already accomplished. Look around, and I'm sure you'll find more than one thing to be proud of. The fact that you have read this book already means that you care enough about yourself to keep improving. Stay present and grounded so that you don't lose yourself in your thoughts. When you feel your thoughts taking over, remember to practice your meditation. Set a reminder on your phone so that you can practice every day. Eventually, it will become a way of life.

The journey to self-discovery is never-ending. As humans, we evolve and change constantly. For this reason, never stop learning about yourself. At times, you might find that what used to make you happy, doesn't anymore. That is okay. It proves the fact you are growing as a person. It also speaks volumes on the fact that your emotional intelligence is maturing. So if you find yourself not craving what you used to, all you have to do is get to know yourself again. When you reach this stage, follow the steps listed in Chapter five of this book to find your happiness again. Don't be afraid to adjust your goals when you evolve. If you grow, then your goals should grow with you. Whatever you do, never give up on your goals just because you are afraid of failing.
Failure is natural and is a part of everyday life. The way you handle your failure defines the kind of person you are. Would you like to be known as the person who gave up in the face of adversity or the person who reached for their goals despite the obstacles? Since you have made it this far, I would like to think of you as the latter. Now, the only thing left to do is to convince yourself of the person you would like to be. Always remember to use a bad experience as a learning curve and improve from there. Even if you do succeed, never stop trying to improve yourself. Allow yourself the courtesy to feel emotions when being confronted by critics. The one thing you should never do is allow your emotions to control. In fact, nothing and no one else should be able to control you, but you.

Life is a journey, one I believe deserves to be explored in its entirety. However, be careful not to take on more than you can handle. No matter how small a step you take, or how slow you travel, I want you to know that it is enough. The only time you're not doing enough is when you're doing nothing at all.

I have provided you with the tools needed to be self-motivated and self-sufficient. I have told you the secret to finding your happiness and setting goals that you want to achieve. I've provided you with the information you need to effectively deal with failure and rid yourself of fear. It is now up to you to use the knowledge of this book to improve yourself and get out of your comfort zone. While navigating this harsh world, I want you to make yourself a priority by being kind, loving, and respectful to yourself. Once you have mastered the art of self-love, I want you to extend that courtesy to everyone you meet in life. Never base your treatment of people based on what they have or don't have. Treat every human with the same kindness and respect that you deserve.

As you begin your journey, I wish you nothing but good luck, prosperity, and success. May you achieve everything that you aim for and may overcome every obstacle in your path. Always remember - you are capable, you are strong, and you are enough.

References

5 Signs You Have A Scarcity Mindset. (2015, November 18) Power of Positivity: Positive Thinking & Attitude. https://www.powerofpositivity.com/5-signs-you-have-a-scarcity-mindset/

6 Reasons Why Failure Is As Equally Important As Success. (2017, November 3). Pick the Brain | Motivation and Self Improvement. https://www.pickthebrain.com/6-reasons-failure-equally-important-success/#:~:text=With%20every%20small%20or%20big

Bradberry, T. (n.d.). *8 Ways Smart People Use Failure To Their Advantage.* Forbes. https://www.forbes.com/sites/travisbradberry/2016/04/12/8-ways-smart-people-use-failure-to-their-advantage/?sh=3bfcd2ab4489

Castrillon, C. (2020, January 19). *5 Healthy Ways To Deal With Criticism At Work.* Forbes. https://www.forbes.com/sites/carolinecastrillon/2020/01/19/5-healthy-ways-to-deal-with-criticism-at-work/?sh=b533048312a4.

Cherry, K. (2010, July 20). *What Exactly Is Self-Esteem?* Verywell Mind; Verywellmind. https://www.verywellmind.com/what-is-self-esteem-2795868

Eric. (2019, March 5). *Benefits of Living with an Abundance Mindset.* The Mastermind Within. https://www.themastermindwithin.com/give-shall-receive-live-abundance-mindset/

Francis, C. A. (2013, April 19). *How to Live in the Moment and Stop Worrying About the Future.* Lifehack. https://www.lifehack.org/articles/communication/21-instant-ways-to-live-in-the-moment.html

Improving Self-Esteem | Skills You Need. (2011) Skillsyouneed. www.skillsyouneed.com/ps/self-esteem.html.

Philippou, T. (2019, August 14). *We have plenty of time. Stop thinking you don't have enough.* Medium. https://medium.com/swlh/we-have-plenty-of-time-stop-thinking-you-dont-have-enough-6c11e33eb82

Pietrzak, M. (2019, September 11). *Want to Be a Leader? Lead Yourself First.* SUCCESS. https://www.success.com/lead-yourself-first/

Rebecca. (2020, June 10). *15 Valuable Ways to Appreciate What You Have*. Minimalism Made Simple. https://www.minimalismmadesimple.com/home/appreciate-what-you-have/

Russ, A. (2020, October 11). *Abundance Mindset*. AGL. https://a-good-life.org/2020/10/11/abundance-mindset/

Sargent, D. (n.d.). *Living in the Light: A guide to personal transformation by David Sargent - PDF Drive*. Pdfdrive. https://www.pdfdrive.com/living-in-the-light-a-guide-to-personal-transformation-e10172273.html

Seredich, B. (2017, December 20). *Why Self-Esteem Is Critical to Successful Leadership*. Engage Blog. https://www.achievers.com/blog/self-esteem-critical-successful-leadership/

The Benefits of Being Grateful That You May Not Know About. (n.d.). Happify. https://www.happify.com/hd/benefits-of-being-grateful-that-you-may-not-know-about/#:~:text=power%20of%20gratitude.

Vedantam, S. (2019). *NPR Choice*. NPR. https://www.npr.org/2017/03/23/5211959 03/how-the-scarcity-mindset-can-make-problems-worse.

www.ingramcontent.com/pod-product-compliance
Lightning Source LLC
Chambersburg PA
CBHW051218250726
48655CB00006B/2471